PRAGATI KHANORKAR
Manju Chandankhede



# Dyslipdemia in Diabetic Retinopathy & Cataract: A Monograph

## A Perspective on Biochemical Parameters

LAP LAMBERT Academic Publishing

**Imprint**


Cover image: www.ingimage.com

Publisher:
LAP LAMBERT Academic Publishing
is a trademark of
Dodo Books Indian Ocean Ltd. and OmniScriptum S.R.L publishing group

120 High Road, East Finchley, London, N2 9ED, United Kingdom
Str. Armeneasca 28/1, office 1, Chisinau MD-2012, Republic of Moldova, Europe
Managing Directors: Ieva Konstantinova, Victoria Ursu
info@omniscriptum.com

Printed at: see last page
**ISBN: 978-620-6-14981-1**

PRAGATI KHANORKAR
Manju Chandankhede

# Dyslipdemia in Diabetic Retinopathy & Cataract: A Monograph

# Dyslipdemia in Diabetic Retinopathy & Cataract: A Monograph

## A Perspective on Biochemical Parameters

# ACKNOWLEDGMENT

I deeply acknowledge the blessings of almighty for giving me the sense for doing my work with sincerity and enthusiasm. Also the love of my late parents boosts me overcome all the obstacles in shaping my work. I cannot repay in words or in deeds the inflable love, moral support to my husband Dr. Prashant Peshattiwar without whom this work would not be in present shape. My little angel master sagar always inspires me to strive for putting my best foot forward.

# Index


| Sr. No. | Title | Page No. |
|---|---|---|
| 1 | Introduction | 9 |
| 2 | Pathophysiology of Diabetic Retinopathy and Cataract | 13 |
| 3 | Diabetic Retinopathy and serum lipids, serum creatinine and serum albumin | 16 |
| 4 | Diabetic Cataract and serum lipids, serum creatinine and serum albumin | 22 |
| 5 | Clinical study | 24 |
| 6 | Discussion | 33 |
| 7 | Conclusion and future trends | 35 |

List of Tables


| Sr. No. | Title | Page no. |
| --- | --- | --- |
| 1 | Blood Parameters for cases and controls | 25 |
| 2 | Age wise distribution between cases and controls | 26 |
| 3 | Gender wise distribution between cases and controls | 26 |
| 4 | Duration of DM with retinopathy and cataract | 27 |
| 5 | Different biochemical parameters among groups | 28 |
| 6 | Blood glucose levels among groups | 29 |
| 7 | Lipid profile parameters among groups | 31 |
| 8 | Serum albumin and serum creatinine among groups | 33 |

# List of Abbreviations:

| | | |
|---|---|---|
| AD | - | After Death of Christ |
| ADA | - | American Diabetes Association |
| AGE | - | Advanced Glycosylated End products |
| AR | - | Aldose Reductase |
| BC | - | Before Christ |
| CRP | - | C Reactive Protein |
| CSME | - | Clinically Significant Macular Oedema |
| Hb | - | Haemoglobin |
| HbA1c | - | Glycosylated haemoglobin |
| HDL | - | High Density Lipoprotein |
| HDL-C | - | High Density Lipoprotein Cholesterol |
| IDF | - | International Diabetes Federation |
| IRMA | - | Intra Retinal Microvascular Abnormalities |
| LDL | - | Low Density Lipoprotein |
| LDL-C | - | Low Density Lipoprotein Cholesterol |
| LOCS | - | Lenticular Opacity Classification System |
| ME | - | Macular Oedema |
| NDR | - | No Diabetic Retinopathy |

| | | |
|---|---|---|
| NPDR | - | Non Proliferative Diabetic Retinopathy |
| NVD | - | Neovascularisation on disc of retina |
| NVE | - | Neovascularisation elsewhere (i.e. other than disc) |
| PDR | - | Proliferative Diabetic Retinopathy |
| T2DM | - | Type 2 Diabetes Mellitus |
| TC | - | Total Cholesterol |
| TG | - | Triglycerides |
| UV | - | Ultra Violet |
| VEGF | - | Vascular Endothelial Growth Factor |
| VLDL | - | Very Low-Density Lipoprotein |
| WHO | - | World Health Organisation |

ABSTRACT

Diabetes with its complications becomes a major cause of blindness worldwide. Diabetic retinopathy and cataract are among its complications. Large number of clinical studies have shown variable results regarding association of serum lipid levels as a risk factor for DR. A study was conducted to find out the role of serum lipids in the development of diabetic retinopathy and cataract in type II Diabetes Mellitus.

One hundred twenty diabetic subjects aged 40-70 years attending OPD at a tertiary centre participated in the study. They were compared with 120 age and sex matched healthy subjects. Subjects were divided into three groups. Group I included diabetic subjects with cataract and no retinopathy. Group II included diabetic subjects with diabetic retinopathy no cataract and Group III included diabetics with retinopathy and cataract both. Fasting blood glucose, post meal blood glucose, HbA1C, serum Triglyceride, Total cholesterol, High density cholesterol (HDL), Low density lipoprotein (LDL) and Very low density lipoprotein (VLDL), albumin and creatinine measurements were done by ERBA EM-360 Analyser and results were recorded for all patients.

It was found that fasting blood glucose, HbA1C levels were significantly associated with both retinopathy and cataract in diabetic subjects. Also duration of diabetes was significantly associated with diabetic retinopathy subjects. Total cholesterol levels were positively corelated with both diabetic cataract and retinopathy subjects but more so with cataract subjects. Serum triglyceride levels were significantly associated with diabetic retinopathy patients as compared to cataract patients. Levels of LDL cholesterol were significantly associated with cataract subjects as compared with other groups.

This study documented significant association between DR and cataract with dyslipidemia in type 2 diabetic patients. So along with regular blood sugar checkup all Diabetics should get their serum lipids checked up regularly & control them if deranged. Preservation of good vision may be a motivating factor for lowering serum lipids.

**Introduction:**

According to the 2021 report by the IDF, approximately 537 million individuals globally were affected with diabetes, constituting roughly 10.5% of the world's population. This condition incurred healthcare expenditures of $966 billion. Projections indicate a surge in diabetes cases to 783 million by 2045, with associated healthcare costs estimated to surpass $1054 billion[1] . Diabetes mellitus is a group of metabolic disorders of carbohydrate metabolism in which glucose is both underutilized as an energy source and overproduced due to inappropriate gluconeogenesis and glycogenolysis, resulting in hyperglycemia[2] .

Type 2 DM is also known as Noninsulin Diabetes Mellitus. The cause of type 2 DM is multifactorial. Genetic susceptibility plays a crucial role in etiology and manifestation of type 2 DM with roots in the interaction of environmental factors, physical activity, obesity, ethnic, drugs, toxic agents, viral infection & location. The current WHO diagnostic criteria for diabetes is – fasting glucose is more than 126 mg/dl, PP 2 hr blood glucose is more than 200 mg/dl & HbA1C is more than 6.5%[3].

Diabetes increases the risk of many different complications that in general can be divided into macro- and microvascular disease. The macrovascular complications include coronary heart disease and cerebrovascular disease. The microvascular complications include neuropathy, nephropathy and diabetic retinopathy[4]. Diabetic retinopathy progresses from various grades of NPDR to Proliferative Diabetic Retinopathy (PDR) and can lead to irreversible effects such as vision loss if not adequately managed. The SMART India study found that among Indians aged 40 years or older, the prevalence of DR was 12.5%, and the prevalence of vision-threatening DR/PDR was 4% (3.4 to 8.8%)[5].

Hypertension, dyslipidemia, and chronic hyperglycaemia are the main risk factors for DR, as they are linked to the pathogenesis and progression

of this microvascular disease. Others are the duration of diabetes, age, and inadequate glycaemic control[6]. Lipid oxidation in DR mediates oxidative stress and various inflammatory mediators that regulate inflammatory cytokines

like Vascular Endothethial Growth Factor (VEGF). The mitochondrial

damage caused by this may accelerate the death of retinal neurons as well as lens fibres aggravating microvascular damage and retinal degeneration and lens changes in diabetes[7,8].

Diabetic cataract is considered a complication of DM, which affect individuals at younger ages and 2–5 times more frequently than healthy subjects.

Several pathogenetic mechanisms that may precipitate formation of diabetic cataract are as follows -

- increased osmotic stress caused by activation of the polyol pathway,
- non-enzymatic glycation of lens proteins, and

- increased oxidative stress.

All these factors cause liquefaction of the lens protein fibres and increased apoptotic activity of lens fibres leading to opacification of lens i.e. cataract4.

Friedman and L'Esperance coined the term "the renal – retinal syndrome" for concurrent renal and eye diseases resulting from changes occurring in retinal and glomerular arterioles and capillaries due to diabetic microangiopathy[9].

According to Steno hypothesis, albuminuria might reflect a general vascular dysfunction and leakage of albumin and other plasma macromolecules such as low-density lipoproteins into the vessel wall that may lead to inflammatory responses[10]. Hyperglycaemia causes formation of amadori products which in turn leads to glycation of various proteins like albumin so role of serum albumin is implicated in the pathogenesis of both diabetic retinopathy and cataract. Hence serum albumin levels might reflect the diabetic complications[11].

For evaluating the importance of serum lipids, serum creatinine and serum albumin in the development of retinopathy and cataractous changes in type 2 Diabetes mellitus patients and early prevention of complications of T2DM a study was conducted at a tertiary care centre with following aims and objectives

1.To measure and compare the level of glycated hemoglobin and fasting blood glucose in patients with diabetic cataract and diabetic retinopathy with healthy individuals.

2.To elucidate the association of lipid profile in diabetic cataract and diabetic retinopathy.

3.To correlate the level of serum albumin in diabetic cataract and diabetic retinopathy.

4.To study the level of Serum creatinine in diabetic cataract and diabetic retinopathy.

**Pathogenesis of Diabetic Retinopathy and cataract**

**Diabetic Retinopathy:**

Diabetic Retinopathy (DR) is the most common microvascular complication of diabetes and leading cause of acquired blindness. According to American Academy of Ophthalmologists (2016) Retinopathy is divided into three main categories: non-proliferative retinopathy, proliferative retinopathy and diabetic macular oedema. Diabetic retinopathy is clinically characterised by micro aneurysms, haemorrhages, venous beading, cotton wool spots, intra retinal microvascular abnormalities (IRMA) and formation of new proliferative vessels. These retinal abnormalities range from changes not visible on a retinal examination or photo to severe proliferative retinopathy with pathological angiogenesis resulting in fibrovascular proliferation on top of the retina or into the vitreous. Such changes eventually lead to vitreous haemorrhage and tractional retinal detachment[12]. The progressive neuroglial and microvascular damage are also affected by various other factors such as hyperglycaemia, impaired retinal autoregulation, dyslipidaemia and impaired renal function. To develop the clinical manifestation of diabetic retinopathy inflammation, leucostasis, ischemia and structural alterations are important features[13]. Histopathological studies of diabetic retinopathy show thickening of the capillary basement membrane, loss of pericytes, micro aneurysms, endothelial cell death and capillary loss[14,15].

a) Loss of pericytes:

Pericytes have contractile properties to control vessel calibre and hence the blood flow. With the loss of pericytes vessels become rigid and the endothelium of the vessel wall is damaged by the increased shear stress. Destruction of the endothelial cells and increased basement membrane thickness, leads to a breakdown of the blood-retina barrier, increasing the permeability of vessel walls to proteins and other substances[16].

b) micro aneurysms:

The response to non-perfusion in some capillaries results in dilation of others. These new vessels are lined with endothelium which has increased permeability. Micro aneurysms are the first feature of DR to become visible on clinical examination[16].

c) Haemorrhages:

As the vessels in micro aneurysms are very fragile they often bleed forming superficial and flame shaped or deeper and more rounded lesions ('blot') haemorrhages. They are frequently associated with small hard exudates, which are an accumulation of plasma lipoprotein[17].

d) Cotton wool spots:

As ischaemia increases, the number of haemorrhages increase and evidence of focal ischaemia in the form of Cotton Wool Spots (CWS) may appear which are infarctions of the retinal nerve fibre layer[18].

**Diabetic cataract:**

Cataract refers to any opacity of the natural crystalline lens that degrades the optical quality. Histopathologically, posterior subcapsular cataract are most commonly seen in Diabetic patients. Posterior sub-capsular cataracts are due to the migration and enlargement of lens epithelial cells (Wedl cells) posteriorly. Complicated cataracts are most commonly seen in diabetic cases with anterior segment complications like pupillary block, posterior synechiae, pigmented precipitates on implants and severe iritis which make the extraction surgery difficult. Some posterior segment complications associated are macular edema, proliferative retinopathy, tractional retinal detachment[19].

# DIABETIC RETINOPATHY

NORMAL RETINA

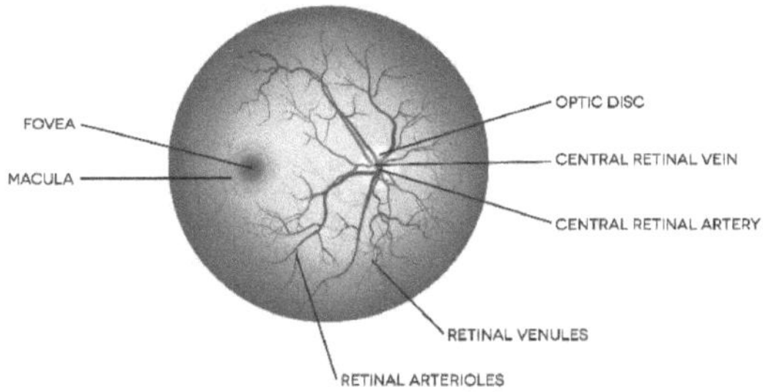


DIABETIC RETINOPATHY

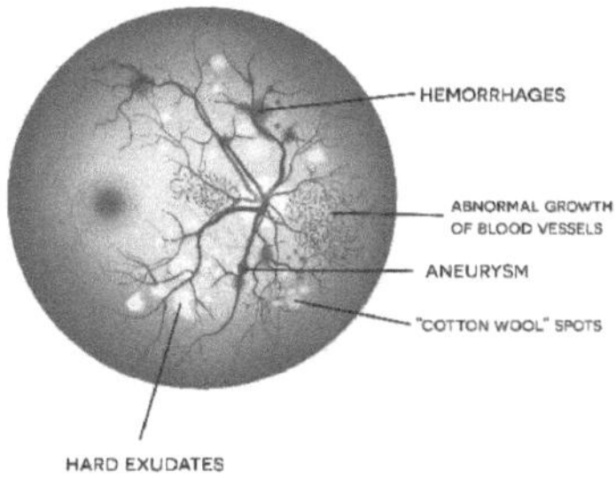


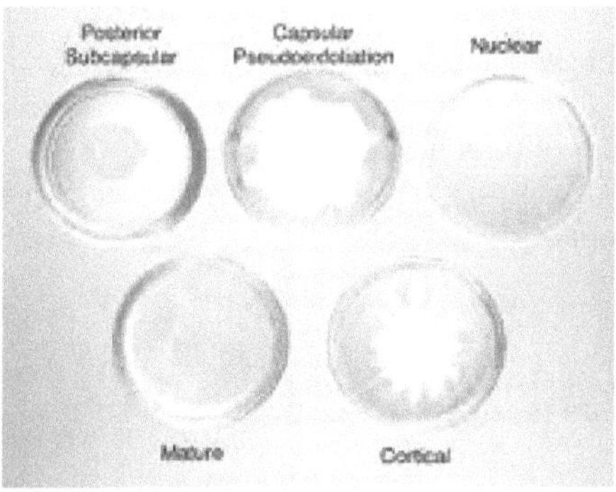


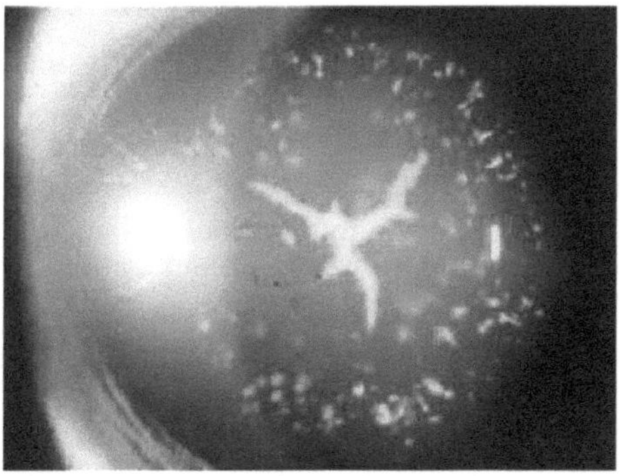

**Diabetic Retinopathy and role of serum lipids, albumin and creatinine**

Pathological mechanisms involved are

1. Hyperglycemia-

   It causes activation of Aldose reductase–mediated polyol pathway, Hexosamine pathway, Protein kinase C activation, Advanced Glycosylated End Products (AGEs)[20] thus leading to pathological changes.

2. Role of lipids –

   Insulin inhibits adipocyte hormone-sensitive lipase and activates lipoprotein lipase. Role of 5 lipo-oxygenase enzyme metabolite in endothelial cell proliferation and angiogenesis of diabetic retinopathy is suggested[21]. Oxidized and glycated LDL induce retinal pericyte apoptosis leading to increased vascular permeability in diabetic retina[22]. Role of glycated phospholipids is also implicated in angiogenesis of diabetic retinopathy[23].

3. Role of albumin-

   Role of reduced form of albumin is suggested to increase vascular permeability in cases of diabetic retinopathy. Albumin competes with other proteins for glycation and low serum albumin level is associated with increased plasma protein glycation, increased fibrinogen glycation in diabetes[24]. It has also been suggested that low plasma albumin predicts the glycated hemoglobin (HbA1c) in type 2 diabetes mellitus.

4. Role of creatinine-

   Skeletal muscle is the most important site of insulin resistance and accounts for approximately 90% of overall glucose disposal after glucose infusion. Systemic markers of inflammation and endothelial dysfunction associated with retinal vascular abnormalities could contribute to the development of kidney disease[25].

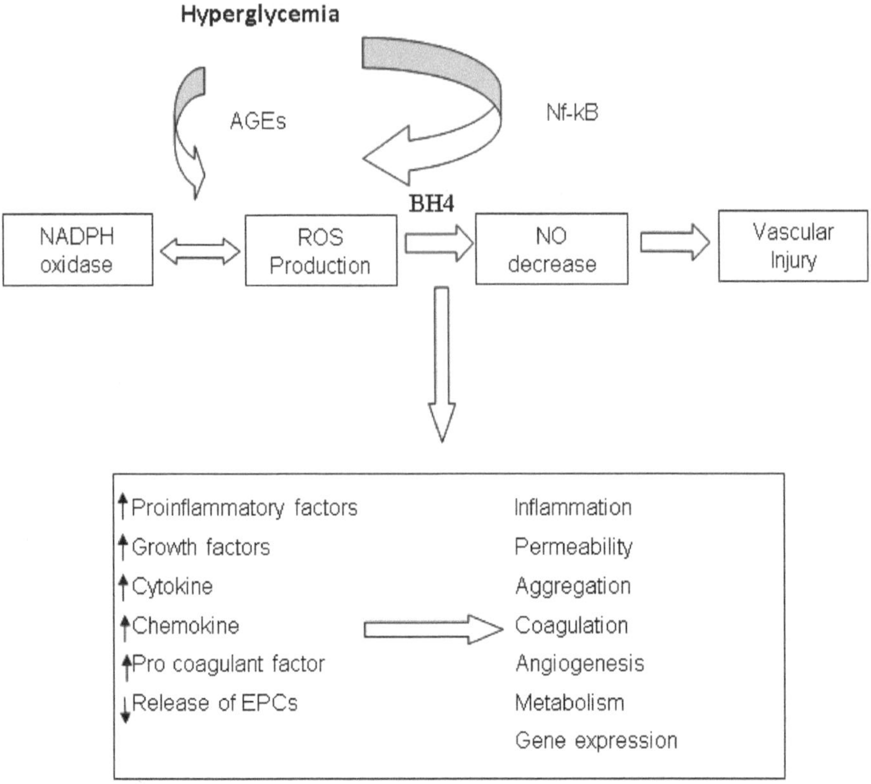


***Critical role of Hyperglycaemia in retinopathy*** Hyperglycaemia plays a central role in states of diabetes mellitus. pathways triggered by advanced glycated end products and mediated by the nuclear factor (Nf)- kB lead to increased oxidative status and thus to impaired nitric oxide (NO) productions/bioavailability. As a result, numerous substances are increased, such as growth factor, cytokines, pro-coagulant factors, and others strongly related to altered underlying processes that induce and promote retinopathy. AGE = Advanced Glycated end product; NADPH = Nicotinamide Adenine Dinucleotide Phosphate, ROS = Reactive Oxygen Species, EPC = Endothelial Progenitor Cell; BH4 = Tetrahydrobiopterin.

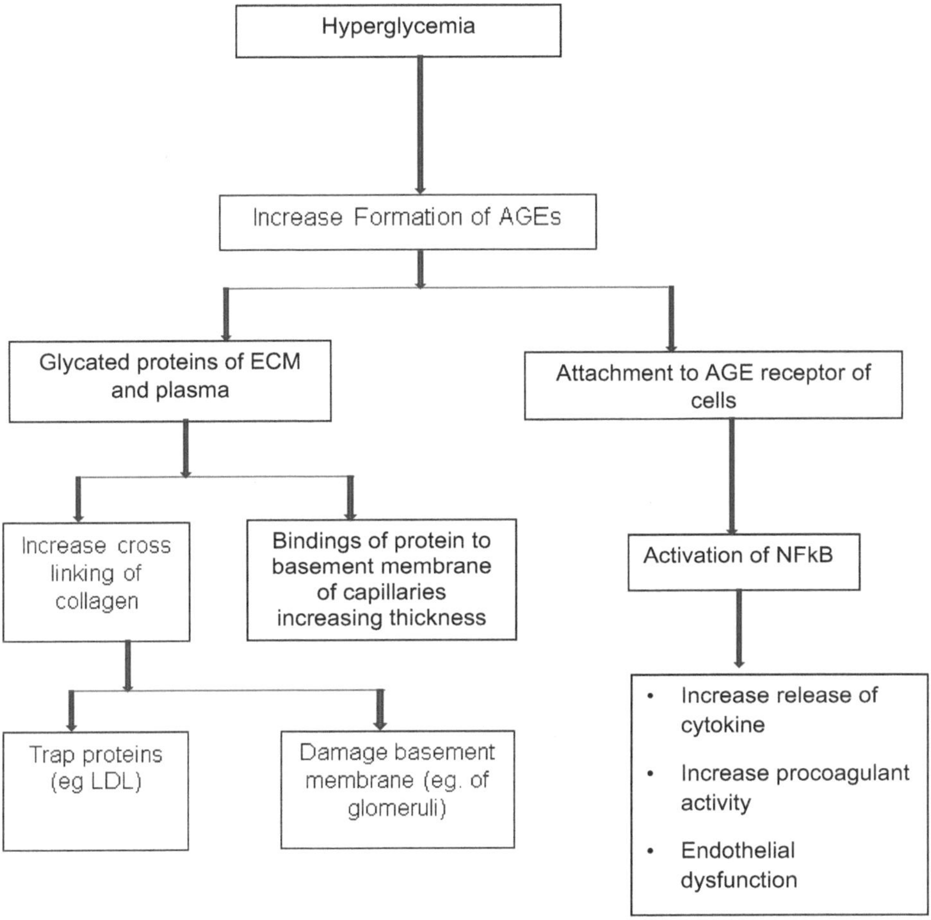


**Some consequences of the formation of advanced glycation end-products**. AGEs = Advanced Glycation End-Products; ECM = Extra Cellular Membrane, NFkB = Nuclear Factor kB; LDL = Low Density Lipoprotein.

**Diabetic Cataract and role of serum lipids, albumin and creatinine**

Cataract is associated with the gradual reduction of visual quality and series of pathways for its development are given as below -

1. Hyperglycaemia Related –

Polyol pathway - The intracellular increase of fluid due to accumulation of polyols results in lens swelling associated with complex biochemical changes ultimately leading to cataract formation[26]. Oxidative stress, Formation of AGEs, Loss of antioxidants also play a major role for the development of cataract.

2. Role of Lipids:

Cholesterol is present in large amount (approximately 40% of the total lipids) in normal human lens fibers. So intrinsic or extrinsic factors modifying its level and/or repartition, may alter optical lens properties[27]. Human lens is continuously in a strong photoxidative environment, a chronic exposure to UV light and ozone can lead to the formation of some cholesterol oxide derivatives (also named oxysterols)[28].

3. Role of Serum Albumin:

Albumin was reported to be shifted to oxidized forms in aqueous humor of cataract patients and also by DM[29].

4. Role of Serum Creatinine:

With increasing oxidative stress like glutathione oxidases in diabetes serum creatinine levels may get affected with cataract development[30].

**Clinical study and correlation:**

A cross sectional study was carried out at a tertiary care hospital to study the role of serum lipids, albumin and creatinine in diabetic subjects with retinopathy and cataract in 2016-2017.

After ethical approval 120 diabetic subjects with retinopathy and cataract were compared with 120 healthy age and sex matched individuals for the said parameters. Upon obtaining informed consent from the study subjects (age group 40-70 years of both sexes) they were grouped as

Group I – Diabetic with cataract no retinopathy

Group II - Diabetic with retinopathy and no cataract

Group III – Diabetic with retinopathy and cataract

Among these Diabetics with other complications such as neuropathy; nephropathy; hypertension and other vascular complications, Diabetic patients with any other concurrent chronic disease such as cardiac diseases; thrombotic stroke; etc. and Gestational diabetes mellitus subjects were excluded from the study.

The study design was explained to all the subjects and all were sent for phlebotomy room for venous blood collection in sterile vacutainers. Blood was taken in two vacutainers 5ml in red and 3ml in purple vacutainers.

The blood samples were then run for the following parameters on ERBA 360 analyser -

| No. | PARAMETER | METHOD |
|---|---|---|
| 1. | **HbA1C** | Kit based on immunoturbidimetry method |
| 2. | **Blood Glucose** | Enzymatic method- Glucose Oxidase and Peroxidase- End point |
| 3. | **Serum creatinine** | Modified kinetic method of Jaffe |
| 4. | **Serum albumin** | BCG method |
| 5. | **Serum cholesterol** | Enzymatic cholesterol oxidase and peroxide - End point method |
| 6. | **HDL** | Modified PEG method |
| 7. | **Serum Triglycerides** | GPO- Trinder method |
| 8. | **Serum LDL** | using Friedwald formula<br>LDL = TC – (HDL + TG/5) |
| 9. | **Serum VLDL** | Using Friedewald equation<br>VLDL = 1/5 TG level (that is TG /5) |

All 120 diagnosed cases of T2DM and 120 age and sex matched normal healthy persons samples were subjected to Fasting plasma glucose (FPG), 2 hours post prandial glucose levels (2hPG), serum creatinine, serum albumin, serum cholesterol, serum triglyceride, serum HDL, serum LDL, serum VLDL, serum creatinine. Study subjects were classified as Group 1 – DM with Cataract, Group 2 - DM with Retinopathy and Group 3 – DM with both Cataract and Retinopathy and above parameters were also compared amongst the Groups.

**Results:**

Biochemical parameters were compared by performing unpaired t - test between cases and control. Categorical variables were compared by performing Chi-square test. The biochemical parameters were also compared between the groups by one-way ANOVA test using SPSS 20 software.

$p < 0.05$ was taken as significant(S)

$p < 0.001$ was taken as highly significant (HS)

$p > 0.05$ was taken as non-significant (NS).

**Age wise distribution among cases and controls**

| AGE (YEARS) | CASES | | CONTROL | |
|---|---|---|---|---|
| | Number | Percent | Number | Percent |
| 41-50 | 27 | 22.5 | 28 | 23.33 |
| 51-60 | 53 | 44.16 | 51 | 42.5 |
| 61-70 | 40 | 33.33 | 41 | 34.16 |
| TOTAL | 120 | 100 | 120 | 100 |
| Mean Age (Range) | 57.76 ± 7.30 (40 - 70) | | 56.74 ± 7.27 (40 – 70) | |

**Gender wise distribution among cases and controls**

| Sex | CASES (n=120) | | CONTROLS (n=120) | |
|---|---|---|---|---|
| | Number | % | Number | % |
| Male | 75 | 62.5 | 75 | 62.5 |
| Female | 45 | 37.5 | 45 | 37.5 |
| Total | 120 | 100 | 120 | 100 |

The above table shows both the groups are age and sex matched and there is no significant association for age and gender with disease.

**Association of Duration of DM with Cataract, Retinopathy and Mixed Groups.**

| Duration of DM (in years) | No. of Cataract | No. of Retinopathy | No. of Mixed |
|---|---|---|---|
| 1 - 5 | 17 (42.5%) | 4 (10%) | 3 (7.5%) |
| 6 - 10 | 15 (37.5%) | 8 (20%) | 10 (25%) |
| 11 - 15 | 5 (12.5%) | 12 (30%) | 13 (32.5%) |
| > 15 | 3 (7.5%) | 16 (40%) | 14 (35%) |

The above table shows the association of retinopathy with the duration of DM. With the increase in the duration of DM there were more chances of retinopathy to the DM patients.

**Different Biochemical Parameters Between Cases and Controls**

| PARAMETERS | CASES (n = 120)<br>MEAN ± SD | CONTROLS (n = 120)<br>MEAN ± SD | P VALUE |
|---|---|---|---|
| FASTING BLOOD GLUCOSE (mg/dl) | 191.03 ± 68.78 | 98.03 ± 7.67 | P<0.001 HS |
| HbA1c | 8.58 ± 1.70 | 5.55 ± 0.55 | p < 0.001 HS |
| SERUM TOTAL CHOLESTEROL (mg/dl) | 264.59 ± 47.52 | 188 ± 17.32 | P< 0.001 HS |
| SERUM TRIGLYCERIDES (mg/dl) | 226.12 ± 41.45 | 145.31 ± 13.85 | P < 0.001 HS |
| SERUM LDL (mg/dl) | 191.64 ± 31.36 | 115.70 ± 18.72 | P < 0.001 HS |
| SERUM VLDL (mg/dl) | 45.210 ± 8.303 | 29.062 ± 2.771 | P <0.001 HS |
| SERUM HDL (mg/dl) | 37.76 ± 4.22 | 43.62 ± 6.52 | P<0.001 HS |
| SERUM CREATININE (mg/dl) | 1.086 ± 0.32 | 0.88 ± 0.28 | P < 0.001 HS |
| SERUM ALBUMIN (gm/dl) | 3.56 ± 0.50 | 4.153 ± 0.52 | P < 0.01 HS |

Table shows diabetics have dyslipidemia, raised creatinine and low albumin levels as compared with the control group showing their progression for complications.

The below shows fasting blood glucose and HbA1C levels are strongly associated with diabetic complications like diabetic cataract and retinopathy.

## Blood Glucose and HbA1c Among Different Groups

| PARAMETER | GROUP | MEAN | F VALUE | p VALUE | MULTIPLE COMPARISONS | t VALUE | p VALUE |
|---|---|---|---|---|---|---|---|
| FPG | 1 | 98.03 | 143.3 | p < 0.0001 | 1 VS 2 | 6.12 | p < 0.001 |
| | 2 | 143.2 | | | 1 VS 3 | 12.55 | p < 0.001 |
| | 3 | 190.7 | | | 2 VS 3 | 5.24 | p < 0.001 |
| | 4 | 239.2 | | | 2 VS 4 | 10.61 | p < 0.001 |
| PMPG | 1 | 118.2 | 186.1 | P <0.0001 | 1 VS 2 | 7.944 | p < 0.001 |
| | 2 | 180.1 | | | 1 VS 3 | 14.38 | p < 0.001 |
| | 3 | 230.3 | | | 2 VS 3 | 5.25 | p < 0.001 |
| | 4 | 287.6 | | | 2 VS 4 | 11.26 | p < 0.001 |
| HbA1c | 1 | 5.51 | 238.8 | p < 0.0001 | 1 vs 2 | 12.04 | p < 0.001 |
| | 2 | 7.68 | | | 1 vs 3 | 17.28 | p < 0.001 |
| | 3 | 8.63 | | | 2 vs 3 | 4.273 | p = 0.001 |
| | 4 | 9.79 | | | 2 vs 4 | 9.53 | p < 0.001 |

1= CONTROL, 2 = CATARACT, 3 = RETINOPATHY, 4 = MIXED

## Blood Glucose Levels in Different Groups

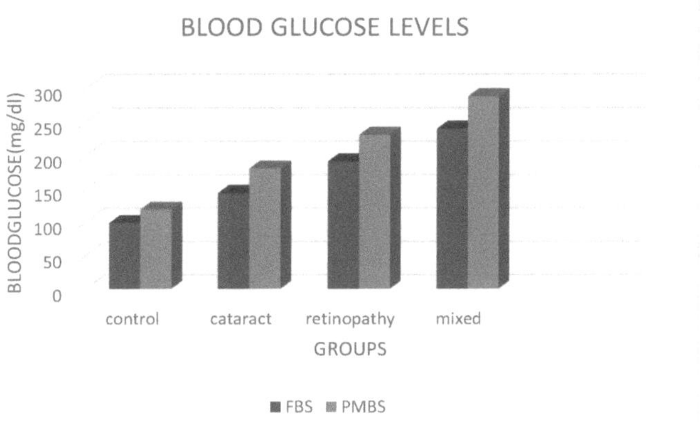

## Lipid Profile in Different Groups

| PARAMETER | GROUP | MEAN | F VALUE | p VALUE | MULTIPLE COMPARISONS | t VALUE | p VALUE |
|---|---|---|---|---|---|---|---|
| TC | 1 | 188.4 | 301 | P <0.0001 | 1 vs 2 | 20.41 | p < 0.001 |
| | 2 | 268.9 | | | 1 vs 3 | 16.33 | p < 0.001 |
| | 3 | 252.9 | | | 2 vs3 | 3.325 | p = 0.04 |
| | 4 | 287.7 | | | 2 vs 4 | 3.876 | p = 0.006 |
| TG | 1 | 145.3 | 290.1 | p < 0.0001 | 1 vs 2 | 12.74 | p < 0.001 |
| | 2 | 192.7 | | | 1 vs 3 | 18.01 | P < 0.001 |
| | 3 | 212.3 | | | 2 vs 3 | 4.303 | p = 0.001 |
| | 4 | 245 | | | 2 vs 4 | 11.48 | p < 0.001 |
| LDL | 1 | 115.7 | 222.1 | p < 0.0001 | 1 vs 2 | 18.11 | p < 0.001 |
| | 2 | 193.9 | | | 1 vs 3 | 13.11 | p < 0.001 |
| | 3 | 172.3 | | | 2 vs 3 | 4.077 | p = 0.002 |
| | 4 | 208.7 | | | 2 vs 4 | 2.804 | p = 0.021 |
| HDL | 1 | 43.62 | 21.29 | p < 0.0001 | 1 vs 2 | 6.6 | p < 0.001 |
| | 2 | 36.55 | | | 1 vs 3 | 5.17 | p < 0.001 |
| | 3 | 38.08 | | | 2 vs 3 | 1.16 | NS |
| | 4 | 38.4 | | | 2 vs 4 | 1.41 | NS |
| VLDL | 1 | 29.06 | 289.7 | p < 0.0001 | 1 vs 2 | 12.68 | p < 0.001 |
| | 2 | 38.5 | | | 1 vs 3 | 18 | p < 0.001 |
| | 3 | 42.46 | | | 2 vs 3 | 4.34 | p < 0.001 |
| | 4 | 48.99 | | | 2 vs 4 | 11.52 | p < 0.001 |
| LDL/ HDL | 1 | 2.703 | 124.4 | p < 0.0001 | 1 vs 2 | 14.23 | p < 0.001 |
| | 2 | 5.45 | | | 1 VS 3 | 10.53 | p < 0.001 |
| | 3 | 4.73 | | | 2 VS 3 | 3.01 | p=0.011 |
| | 4 | 5.65 | | | 2 VS 4 | 0.87 | NS |

## TC, TG, and LDL Values in Different Groups

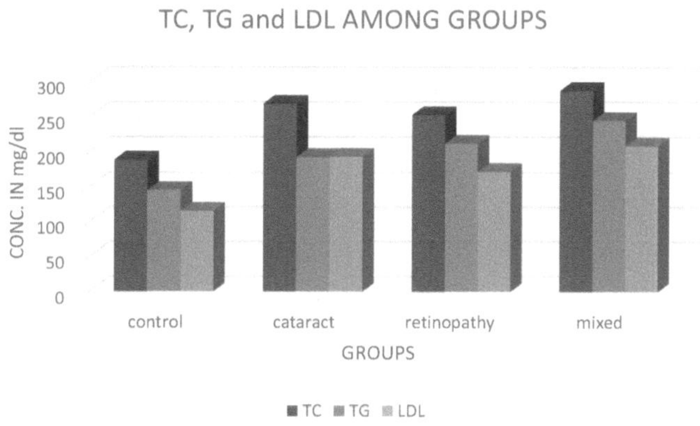


This table compares the lipid profile among different groups. Serum total cholesterol is significantly associated ($p<0.001$) with cataract development as against the retinopathy.

Serum triglycerides are significantly raised ($p<0.001$) among all the groups but more with retinopathy as compared to cataract group ($p=0.001$).

Serum LDL is significantly raised ($P<0.001$) in cataract group as compared to retinopathy ($p<0.05$) group.

Serum LDL/HDL ratio is significantly raised ($p<0.05$) in cataract group which is non-significant for the retinopathy group.

## Sr. Creatinine and Sr. Albumin Levels in Different Groups

| PARAMETER | GROUP | MEAN | F VALUE | p VALUE | MULTIPLE COMPARISONS | t VALUE | p VALUE |
|---|---|---|---|---|---|---|---|
| SR. CREATININE | 1 | 0.88 | 10.3 | p < 0.0001 | 1 VS 2 | 1.382 | NS |
| | 2 | 0.94 | | | 1 VS 3 | 5.04 | p < 0.001 |
| | 3 | 1.10 | | | 2 VS 3 | 2.98 | p=0.012 |
| | 4 | 1.03 | | | 2 VS 4 | 1.73 | NS |
| SR. ALBUMIN | 1 | 4.153 | 30.73 | p < 0.0001 | 1 vs 2 | 5.716 | p < 0.001 |
| | 2 | 3.63 | | | 1 vs 3 | 7.021 | p < 0.001 |
| | 3 | 3.51 | | | 2 vs 3 | 1.06 | NS |
| | 4 | 3.48 | | | 2 vs 4 | 1.37 | NS |

1= CONTROL, 2 = CATARACT, 3 = RETINOPATHY, 4 = MIXED

This table suggests serum creatinine is significantly associated (p<0.001) with retinopathy development but no such association is for cataract development.

There is no relation of serum albumin in cataract and retinopathy development.

**Discussion:**

In this study, Maximum subjects in diabetic group were found in the age group of 51-60 years. Age, body habitus and physical activity all play a role in the pathogenesis of hyperglycaemia associated with diabetes mellitus. Also the positive correlation of retinopathy with the duration of DM was shown which corresponds with the, Katulanda et al, 2014[31].

In present study, serum triglycerides were significantly raised in cataract ($p<0.001$), retinopathy ($p<0.001$) groups when compared with controls. But retinopathy group has shown significant rise ($p=0.001$) as compared to cataract group. suggesting role of serum triglycerides for the raised oxidative stress responsible for retinopathy changes. Also total cholesterol was significantly raised ($p<0.001$) in diabetic patients as compared to control group but there is significant rise ($p<0.05$) in cataract patients as compared to retinopathy. Thus, it suggests major role of serum cholesterol levels with the development of cataract as compared to retinopathy. Similar observation was done by Heydari et al 2012[32] suggesting the role of oxysterol, an oxidative derivative of cholesterol for raised oxidative stress leading to cataract formation. In the present study, serum LDL ($p<0.001$) significantly raised ($p<0.05$) in cataract patients as compared to retinopathy patients.

All these suggests hyperlipidemia in severe DR leads to endothelial dysfunction, resulting in the collapse of the blood-retinal barrier and causing lipids to leak from injured retinal capillaries. This contributes to retinal oedema and the accumulation of hard exudates in the retina[33]. Seema KS et al. has shown that there was a statistically significant association between serum lipid levels and hyperglycaemia across the severity of DR, which increased from mild to severe NPDR and PDR[34]. Similar results are seen in this study, we found a direct and significant association between retinopathy and FBG ($p<0.001$) and PMBG ($p<0.001$). Sachdev and Sahni study[35] in North India documented significant correlation between retinal hard exudates and systolic blood pressure, TC, LDL-C, and TG levels.

In present study, serum creatinine level is significantly raised ($p<0.05$) in retinopathy patients whereas no such relation was found for cataract patients.

**Conclusion:**

Lipid profile, serum creatinine, serum albumin are analysed in both diabetic retinopathy and cataract group verses healthy controls. Among the lipid profile serum triglycerides, serum cholesterol are associated with retinopathy changes. Serum creatinine is positively associated with the retinopathy changes. Diabetic cataract is more strongly associated with serum cholesterol as compared to retinopathy. Also, diabetic cataract is positively associated with serum LDL and LDL/HDL ratio and not with serum creatinine and serum albumin. Both diabetic retinopathy and cataract are positively associated with blood glucose, HbA1c levels.

These results demonstrate the importance of monitoring lipid levels at each stage of retinopathy for effective treatment and help avoid further complications of dyslipidemia in patients with retinopathy as well as cataract. Thus, controlling lipid parameters and blood glucose may retard the retinopathy and cataract changes in type 2 DM patients.

**Future Trends:**

As the results of studies regarding the relationship between lipid profile and retinopathy were inconsistent, it is suggested that more research on lipidemia-induced regulation of circulating biomarkers associated with the degree of DR is needed to predict dyslipidemia at its early stage.

**References:**


1. Hossain MJ, Al-Mamun M, Islam MR. Diabetes mellitus, the fastest growing global public health concern: Early detection should be focused. Health Sci Rep. 2024 Mar 22;7(3):e2004. doi: 10.1002/hsr2.2004. PMID: 38524769; PMCID: PMC10958528.

2. Sacks DB, Arnold M, Bakris GL, et al. Guidelines and recommendations for laboratory analysis in the diagnosis and management of diabetes mellitus. Diabetes Care 2023;46:e151–e199

3. American Diabetes Association. Diabetes Care. 2011 Jan; 34(Suppl 1): S62–S69.

4. Marshall SM, Flyvbjerg Prevention and early detection of vascular complications of diabetes. A BMJ.2006;333:475– 480.

5. Raman R, Vasconcelos JC, Rajalakshmi R, Prevost AT, Ramasamy K, Mohan V, et al. SMART India Study Collaborators. Prevalence of diabetic retinopathy in India stratified by known and undiagnosed diabetes, urban-rural locations, and socioeconomic indices: Results from the SMART India population-based crosssectional screening study. Lancet Glob Health. 2022;10(12):e1764-e1773. Doi:10.1016/S2214-109X(22)00411-9.

6. Vujosevic S, Aldington SJ, Silva P, Hernández C, Scanlon P, Peto T, Simó R. Screening for diabetic retinopathy: New perspectives and challenges. Lancet Diabetes Endocrinol. 2020;8(4):337-47. Doi: 10.1016/S2213-8587(19)30411-5.

7. Rübsam A, Parikh S, Fort PE. Role of inflammation in diabetic retinopathy. Int J Mol Sci. 2018;19(4):942. https://doi.org/10.3390/ijms19040942.

8. Yang C, Xie L, Gu Q, Qiu Q, Wu X, Yin L. 7-Ketocholesterol disturbs RPE cells phagocytosis of the outer segment of photoreceptor and induces inflammation through ERK signaling pathway. Exp Eye Res. 2019;189:107849. Doi: 10.1016/j.exer.2019.107849

9. Friedman EA and L'Esperance FA (Eds): Diabetic Renal-Retinal Syndrome. New York: Grune and Stratton. 1980.

10. Deckert T, Feldt-Rasmussen B, Borch-Johnsen K, et al. Albuminuria reflects widespread vascular damage. The Steno hypothesis. Diabetologia 1989; 32:219-226.

11. Rondeau P, Bourdon E. The glycation of albumin: structural and functional impacts. Albumin is sensitive for glycation because of high half-life and high concentration as compared to other plasma proteins Biochimic 2011; 93: 645 – 658.

12. Ciulla TA, Harris A, Latkany P, Piper HC, Arend O, Garzozi H, Martin B: Ocular perfusion abnormalities in diabetes. Acta Ophthalmol Scand 2002, 80(5):468-477.

13. Ola MS, Nawaz MI, Siddiquei MM, Al-Amro S, Abu El-Asrar AM: Recent advances in understanding the biochemical and molecular mechanism of diabetic retinopathy. J Diabetes Complications 2012, 26(1):56-64.

14. Curtis TM, Gardiner TA, Stitt AW: Microvascular lesions of diabetic retinopathy: clues towards understanding pathogenesis[quest]. Eye 2009, 23(7):1496-1508.

15. Ciulla TA, Harris A, Latkany P, Piper HC, et al: Ocular perfusion abnormalities in diabetes. Acta Ophthalmol Scand 2002, 80(5):468-477.

16. Kohner EM Diabetic retinopathy BMJ. 1993 Nov 6;307(6913):1195-9.

17. Cunha-Vaz J. Photocoagulation for macular edema and proliferative retinopathy. 2010. Chapter 7 Pages 211-236 in Gomez-Ulla F, ed. Diabetic Retinopathy, World Scientific Publishing Co. Diabetic Retinopathy.

18. Early Treatment Diabetic Retinopathy Study Research Group. 1991a. Early photocoagulation for diabetic retinopathy. ETDRS report number 9. Ophthalmology 98: 766-7.

19. Nuclear Sclerosis Cataract Ophthalmic Epidemiology. 1997;4;195-206.

20. H. Zong, M. Ward, and A. W. Stitt, “AGEs, RAGE, and diabetic retinopathy,” Current Diabetes Reports, vol. 11, no. 4, pp. 244–252, 2011.

21. Sapieha P, Stahl A, et al 5-Lipoxygenase metabolite 4-HDHA is a mediator of the antiangiogenic effect of ω-3 polyunsaturated fatty acids. Sci Transl Med. 2011 Feb 9; 3(69):69ra12.

22. Tserent soodol N, Sztein J, et al Uptake of cholesterol by the retina occurs primarily via a low-density lipoprotein receptor-mediated process Mol Vis. 2006 Oct 27; 12():1306-18.

23. Nakagawa K, Oak JH, Miyazawa T Ann N Y Angiogenic potency of Amadori-glycated phosphatidylethanolamine. Acad Sci. 2005 Jun; 1043():413-6.

24. Bhonsle HS, Korwar AM, Kote SS, Golegaonkar SB, Chougale AD, Shaik ML, et al. Low plasma albumin levels are associated with increased plasma protein glycation and HbA1c in diabetes. J Proteome Res. 2012; 11:1391–6.

25. C. Sabanayagam, A. Shankar, D. Kohetal., “Retinal microvascular calibre and chronic kidney disease in an Asian population,” The American Journal of Epidemiology, 2009, vol.169, no.5, pp.625– 632.

26. Yanoff, Myron; Duker, Jay S. Textbook of Ophthalmology (3rd ed.). Edinburgh: Mosby. 2008, p. 412.

27. Zigman S, Paxhia T, Marinetti G, Girsch S Lipids of human lens fibre cell membranes. Curr Eye Res. 1984 Jul; 3(7):887-96.

28. Dreyfus MA, Tolocka MP, Dodds SM, Dykins J, Johnston MV. Cholesterol ozonolysis: kinetics, mechanism and oligomer products. Journal of Physical Chemistry A. 2005;109(28):6242–6248.

29. Kawai K, Yoh M, Hayashi T, Imai H, Negawa T, Tomida M, Sogami M & Era S Effect of diabetic retinopathy on redox state of aqueous humor and serum albumin in patients with senile cataract. Tokai J Exp Clin Med (2001): 26: 93–99.

30. Mathias R.T., Kistler J., Donaldson P. The lens circulation. J. Membr. Biol. 2007; 216:1–16.

31. Katulanda P, Ranasinghe P, Jayawardena R. Prevalence of retinopathy among adults with self- reported diabetes mellitus: the Srilanka diabetes and cardiovascular study. BMC Ophthalmology 2014, 14(100).

32. B Heydari, TKazemi, AZarban, S Ghahramani Correlation of Cataract with Serum Lipids, Glucose and Antioxidant Activities a Case-control Study West Indian Med J 2012;61(3):230-234.

33. Chou Y, Ma J, Su X, Zhong Y. Emerging insights into the relationship between hyperlipidemia and the risk of diabetic retinopathy. Lipids Health Dis. 2020;19(1):241. Doi: 10.1186/s12944-020-01415-3.

34. Seema KS, Binu SS, Bhaskar MK. An observational study on the association between diabetic retinopathy and serum lipid levels in a tertiary center in Thiruvananthapuram. J Evid Based Med Healthc. 2021;8(03):131-35. Doi: 10.18410/jebmh/2021/25.

35. Sachdev N and Sahni A (2010) Association of systemic risk factors with the severity of retinal hard exudates in a north Indian population with type 2 diabetes. J Postgrad Med 56: 3-6.

FSC
www.fsc.org
MIX
Papier | Fördert gute Waldnutzung
FSC® C083411

Kolibri 360 GmbH
Ferdinand-Jühlke-Straße 7
99095 Erfurt, Deutschland
produktsicherheit@kolibri360.de

Druck:
CPI Druckdienstleistungen GmbH
im Auftrag der
Kolibri 360 GmbH
Ferdinand-Jühlke-Str. 7
99095 Erfurt